CW01664953

Stem Cell

A Hope In Cardiology

By: Bhargav Dave, PT, DPT
Myrtle Oates, MD

Copyright © 2016 by Dr. Bhargav Dave
All rights reserved. This book or any portion thereof
may not be reproduced or used in any manner whatsoever
without the express written permission of the publisher
except for the use of brief quotations in a book review.

Printed in the United States of America

First Printing, Oct 20, 2016

E-Book ISBN 978-0-9981743-2-7
Print Book ISBN 978-0-9981743-3-4

Srinivas University Press

2804 Field Hollow Dr,
Pearland, Texas, USA 77584

ACKNOWLEDGEMENTS

I would like to thank my wife Asmi Dave for all the help and encouragements throughout the journey. I would also like to thank my daughter Myra and Yoyo for filling my life with joy and provided me much needed refuge in desperate times.

I would like to thank Divine Mother and Sri Aurobindo for paving the road ahead and guiding my life.

Sit in meditation! But do not think! Look only at your mind! You will see thoughts coming into it! Before they can enter, throw these away from your mind till your mind is capable of entire silence.

- **Sri Aurobindo**

INDEX

1 Introduction: Basics of Stem Cell Biology

Stem cells are found in multi-cellular organisms. These are the specialized cells and have the following properties (Gardner, 2002; Kumar et al., 2010; Bindu & Srilatha et al., 2011; Satessa et al., 2015);

- Self-renewal: Stem cells have ability to undergo numerous cycles of cell division and maintaining the undifferentiated state.
- Potency: Stem cells have potency to differentiate into other types of cell. Example, if adult stem cells isolated from liver tissue and then re-injected into liver become hepatocytes, and if same cells injected into the myocardium, then it became myocytes.

  Potency includes totipotency, pluripotency, multipotent and unipotent.

Various potencies of stem cells:

- *Totipotent:* These stem cells are produced from the fusion of an egg and sperm cells. Further, cells that are produced by the first few divisions of the fertilized egg also called as totipotent. Totipotent stem cells can give rise to somatic progenitor cells and primitive germ- line stem cells.

- *Pluripotent:* Pluripotent are the descendants of totipotent cells, and it can differentiate into nearly all the cells, e.g. cells derived from any different kind of germ layers: ectoderm, mesoderm, and endoderm, as well as the germ lineage. However, it provides little or no contribution to the trophoblast layers of the placenta. Embryonic stem cells come under this category.
- *Multipotent:* This type of stem cells can produce only cells of a closely related family of cells. (e.g., hematopoietic stem cells which are differentiated into red blood cells, white blood cells, platelets, etc.).
- *Oligopotent:* Such stem cells can differentiate into only a few cells, such as lymphoid or myeloid stem cells.
- *Unipotent:* This perticular type of Stem cells only produce one cell type. They have the property of self-renewal which distinguishes them from non-stem cells (e.g., muscle stem cells).

- Plasticity: It is the property of the stem cells by which they can mix with different cells.

- Stem cells also have the property to reach to the different parts of the body.

Generally, stem cells are stored in niches. These are located deep in the tissue so that it provides protection from damaging stimuli. Various chemical and physical signals modulate the behavior of stem cells. Cell surface adhesion molecules, cytokines, shear forces, oxygen levels/tension and ions are major modulators of stem cell function. Further, various cell to cell signaling and a various modulators mediate promotes self-renewal, favoring their migration and differentiation (Leri et al., 2014).

This chapter provides the overview of the major types of stem cells, both from cardiac or extra-cardiac origins; myocyte turnover, cardiac stem cells under normal homeostatic and in unstable conditions; and about cardiac stem cell therapy.

2 Cardiac Stem Cells (CSC)/Cardiac Progenitor Cells (CPC)

Multipotent stem cells are distributed throughout the heart. Under normal physiological conditions, cardiac stem cells are quiet and do not contribute significantly to myocyte renewal. But after any injury, cardiac stem cells can be activated and then differentiated into new myocytes / vascular cells (Le and Chong, 2016).

Several cardiac stem cells have been reported in the developing and adult heart. E.g., c-Kit+; epicardium-derived cells; Islet-1 (Isl-1+) expressing stem cells, stem cell antigen-1 (Sca-1+), cardiac side population cells and cardiospheres.

2.1 c-Kit+ cardiac stem cells

Among all the resident cardiac stem cells, the c-Kit+ cardiac stem cells population has been thoroughly characterized where the c-Kit is the tyrosine kinase receptor (Akhtar, 2013; van Berlo et al, 2014).

C-Kit(+) cardiac stem cells expressed the genes that are involved in the clone formation and cardiosphere generation. Further, they have the potential to differentiate into the cardio-myocyte, smooth muscle, and endothelial cells. It was reported that c-kit(+) CSCs when co-cultured in adult rat cardio-myocytes, it increased cardio-myocyte survival (Miyamoto, et al. 2010).

Many research articles showed that c-kit[+] cardiac stem cells showed considerable potential for proliferation, differentiation and self-renewal under diverse conditions both *in-vitro* and *in-Vivo* and have the ability to repair damaged heart and improve the cardiac function (Dawn et al., 2005; Beltrami et al., 2003; Akhtar, 2013; van Berlo et al, 2014).

Phase 1 study indicates that, intracoronary infusion of autologous cardiac stem cells (c-kit[+]) is effective in improving left ventricular systolic function and reducing infarct size in patients with heart failure after myocardial infarction. This study raised many questions about the integrity of the data. Thus, further studies will be required for any concluding remark (Bolli et al., 2011; The Lancet, 2014).

2.2 Epicardium-derived cells

Epicardium-derived cells are very essential for cardiac development as it involves the formation of the myocardium, coronary vasculature, and purkinje tissue. These cells also contribute to the fibrous heart skeleton, atrio-ventricular valves (AV valve) and the semilunar (Winter and Gittenberger-de Groot, 2007).

It has been reported that defects/disturbed in epicardium-derived cells lead to the defect in the differentiation of the myocardium and defects in the development of the vascular bed (Gittenberger-de Groot et al., 2010).

Epicardium-derived cells have been explored as a stem cell source in various animal models. Studies have shown that there was improved function, angiogenesis, and decrease adverse results in the animal model of myocardial ischemia. A further combination of epicardium-derived cells and other cardiac stem cell have the synergistically improvement in the cardiac function (Gittenberger-de Groot et al., 2010 and Weeke-Klimp et al., 2010).

2.3 Cardiac side population (CSP) cells

Side population (SP) cells were initially reported to be present in the hematopoietic stem cells of the mouse. Side population cells are present in the organs like heart, brain, liver, lung, bone marrow, skeletal muscle and skin. Side population cells present in the heart has the potential of the differentiation into functional myocyte (Hierlihy et al., 2002; Oyama et al., 2007; Pfister et al., 2008).

During the normal physiological condition, resident cardiac side population cells are mainly involved in the cell proliferation. However, during the MI, a massive damage occurs to the side population cells of the heart. So, side population cells from the distant organs also migrate to the heart. Ideally, within seven days baseline levels of the side population cells is achieved with the proliferation and differentiation of the resident side population cells and conversion of the migrated stem cells to the side population cells (Mouquet et al., 2005).

It has been reported that when *Wnt* signaling down regulated, there was increase proliferation of the side population cells. Further administration of the insulin growth factor (IGF) binding protein, IGFBP3 (IGF binding protein 3) also decrease the proliferation side population cells. Overall, both these factors regulates the side population cell proliferation (Unno et al., 2012).

Side population cell function is also dependent on expression of the ATP-binding cassette transporter. Abcg2 (ABC, super family G, member 2) promotes side population cells proliferation capacity and differentiation capacity. Lastly, they also help cells to survival in the oxidative stress (Unno et al., 2012).

2.4 Cardiospheres

Cardiospheres (CSs) has the clonogenic and self-renewing potential, and they are differentiable into cardio-myocytes, endothelial cells, and smooth muscle cell.

Cardiospheres cells are suitable to grow in the culture where it can expand into many folds as monolayers and thus cells number suitable for therapy can be achieved easily. Animal studies reported that therapy with the cardiospheres cells improves left ventricular ejection fraction (Chimenti et al., 2010).

Li *et al.* performed a comprehensive comparison of different cell types in the same animal model in the same laboratory and blinded analysis. Results showed that cardiospheres derived cells were superior in promoting cardio-myogenic differentiation, angiogenesis, paracrine factor secretion, and ischemic tissue preservation and it also has the functional benefit (Li et al., 2012).

In Cardiosphere-derived autologous Stem Cells to reverse ventricular dysfunction (CADUCEUS) trial, patients with left ventricular ejection fraction of 25–45% were enrolled after 2–4 weeks of myocardial infarction. Study results showed that there were reductions in scar mass; improvement in the regional contractility, and regional systolic wall thickening and increases in heart mass after patients treated with cardiospheres derived cells. Further, intracoronary infusion of these cells was safe (Makkar R et al., 2012).

2.5 **Islet-1+ cardiac stem cells**

There are two populations of the cardiogenic mesoderm. The first population of cardiac progenitors, known as the first heart field can give rise first to the cardiac crescent, linear heart tube, and it contributes to parts of the atrial chambers and the left ventricular region. The second population of cardiac progenitors (called as the second heart field) in which Islet-1 plays as a transcription factor, has the potential to give birth to outflow tract. These cells also contribute to the endothelial and vascular smooth muscle lineages development (Sun et al, 2007; Laugwitz et al., 2008).

Animal studies also have shown that genetic defects in Islet-1+ lead to defect in the self-renewal, differentiation, and lineage specification. It has the crucial role in the development of various cardiac lineages (Moretti et al., 2006).

Few questions about human Islet-1+ stem cells needs to be investigated, e.g. 1. distribution in healthy and diseased heart, 2. relationship between Islet-1+ stem cells and other cardiac stem cell, 3. its therapeutic potentiating in the cardiac failure (Ge et al, 2015).

2.6 Stem cell antigen-1 (Sca-1+) stem cells

Sca-1 is an 18-kDa mouse glycosyl phosphatidylinositol-anchored cell surface protein (GPI-AP) (Holmes and Stanford, 2007).

Animal studies reported that it is present in the hematopoietic, mammary gland, and vascular niche. Sca-1 promotes adhesion, proliferation, cellular differentiation and modulates integrin function. (Bailey et al., 2012).

Various *in-vitro* and *in-vivo* studies showed that cardiac stem cells also express Sca-1. These stem cells are involved in the myocardial contractility, repair and dilated cardiomyopathy as the genetic Sca1 animal model showed impairment in the contractibility and repair (Bailey et al., 2012; Ge et al.,2015).

Injury to myocardial tissue causes the proliferation of the Sca-1+ and also stem cells from the distant organ also migrate to the site of myocardial damage to promote the repair (Orlic et al., 2001, Wang et al., 2006).

3 Extra-cardiac stems cells

Few stem cells from the extra-cardiac origin are also involved in the contractibility and vascularization of the myocardium. The same have been described below:

3.1 Platelet-derived growth factors (PDGFs)

Platelet-derived growth factors (PDGFs) affect various cellular responses, like proliferation, differentiation, migration, and survival. The PDGF family includes PDGF-A, PDGF-B, PDGF-C, and PDGF-D. There are the two PDGF receptors, PDGFR-α and PDGFR-β, to which PDGF bind and activate. These are the tyrosine kinase receptors. PDGF-A, PDGF-B, and PDGF-C binds to the PDGFR-α and PDGF-B and PDGF-D binds to the PDGFR-β. PDGFR-α signaling pathway facilitate the development of cranial neural crest (involve in the development of skeleton of the face), cardiac neural crest (responsible for the development of the cardiac outflow track), gonads, skeleton, lung, intestine, central nervous system, and skin. PDGFR-β signaling pathways facilitate the formation of the blood vessel and have the role in the early hematopoiesis (Pontén et al., 2003; Andrae et al., 2008).

PDGF interaction with its receptors forms receptor heterodimers. This dimerization leads to the auto-phosphorylation of tyrosine residues and its activation (Heldin et al., 2013).

It has been reported that PDGFRα-expressing cells are one of the crucial cardiovascular progenitors capable of multi-lineage differentiation. These cells maintain a mesenchymal and vascular portion of the heart. They also increase the cardiac protein or transcription factors expression (Chong et al., 2013).

3.2 Mesenchymal stem cells (MSC)

These cells are present in adult tissues and can be isolated and expanded in the culture. These cells have the ability to differentiate readily into myocyte, adipocytes, chondrocytes, osteocytes and endothelial cell. Published literature supports that these cells also express phenotypic characteristics of cardiac myocyte cells (Pittenger and Martin, 2004; and Karantalis and Hare, 2015).

MSCs have the property to adhere plastic in cell culture, low immunogenicity, specific surface antigen expression and differentiation ability (Williams et al., 2011; Choi et al., 2011).

MSCs have the crucial role in the immune system (Fig. 1) and have the immunosuppressive activity. This activity is due to secretion of the various soluble factors, such as indoleamine 2,3-dioxygnease, nitric oxide, and heme oxygenase-1 via cell-cell contact with specific immune cells. MSCs inhibit both innate and adaptive immune cells. They have the capability to produce anti-fibrotic factors and matrix metalloproteinase. This also helps in the remodeling of the extracellular matrix (Williams et al., 2011; White et al., 2016).

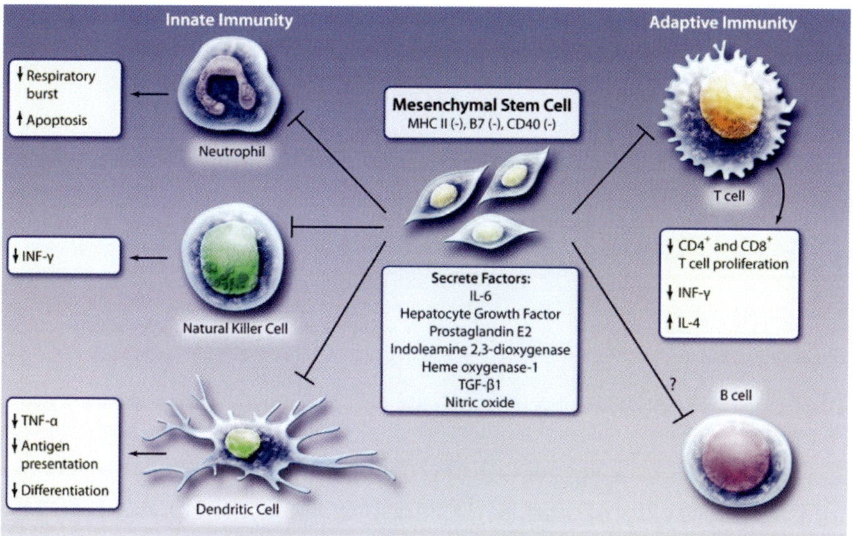

Figure 1: MSC interactions with various immune cells (Williams et al., 2011)**.**

INF-γ indicates interferon-γ; TNF, tumor necrosis factor.

MSCs have the property to induce angiogenesis, reduce fibrosis and restore contractile function of the heart by various paracrine effect and stimulation of cells differentiation as mention in the Fig. 2 (Karantalis and Hare, 2015).

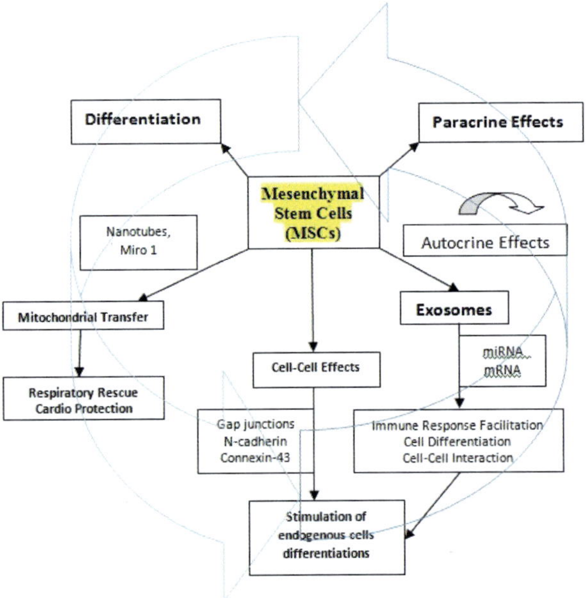

Figure 2: Mechanisms of action of mesenchymal stem cells (MSCs).

The proposed mechanism of action of MSCs forms an intertwined cycle of paracrine, autocrine, and direct effects that include vascular regeneration, myocardial protection, and cardio-myocyte regeneration that ultimately leads to cardiac repair. Miro1 indicates mitochondrial Rho-GTPase.

Various studies (*in-vitro, in-vivo* and clinical trials) support the use of MSC during the MI (Karantalis and Hare, 2015).

In the clinical trials, it has been reported that therapy with MSC improves left ventricular function, the functional capacity of patient, cardiac remodeling and overall quality of life (Hare et al., 2012; Chen et al., 2004; Karantalis et al., 2014).

Clinical trials also showed that there was a 30% to 50% improvement in the MI scar with bone marrow derived MSCs. These will cause restoration of contractile performance and preserved/increase perfusion. Further, therapy of MSCs is safe and feasible (Bartunek et al., 2013; Karantalis and Hare, 2015).

3.3 Skeletal myoblasts cells

Skeletal muscle has the capacity to repair itself after any injury since they contain 'satellite cells' which have the ability to fuse with the muscle fiber and surrounding myoblast to regenerate the skeletal muscle which is functional. However, heart muscle lacks this capacity (Taylor et al., 1998). Pre-clinical studies showed that skeletal myoblast cells improve myocardial performance. Phase I clinical trial showed that skeletal myoblast cell transplantation for the treatment of MI is feasible. However, one study that involves 4-year follows up showed that therapy with skeletal myoblast increase the risk of developing serious arrhythmia and has no positive effect on the heart (Menasché et al., 2003; Veltman et al., 2008).

3.4 Bone marrow mononuclear cells

Bone marrow mononuclear cell therapy is suitable for stem cell therapy due to it contains a hematopoietic and non-hematopoietic cell. It was reported that they may have the property to stimulate paracrine and angiogenesis effect (Laflamme and Murry, 2011; Simari et al., 2014)

Results from many clinical trials have suggested that bone marrow mononuclear cell delivery after acute myocardial infarction (AMI) results in improvement in left ventricular function and is safe. However, few studies also concluded that careful reconsideration should be given to this approach of the therapy (Arnous et al., 2012 and Simari et al., 2014).

3.5 Endothelial stem cells

Endothelial stem cells originate from multiple precursors within the bone marrow and present in different stages of endothelial differentiation in peripheral blood. These cells are positive for both a hematopoietic stem cell marker (e.g., CD34) and an endothelial marker protein (e.g., VEGFR2) (Lee and Poh, 2014).

Endothelial stem cells are present in the bone marrow and are mobilized to the circulation by various stimuli such as certain drugs, ischemia, and exercise training. These cells are involved in the endothelial cell layer maintenance (Möbius-Winkler et al., 2009).

Endothelial plays a crucial role in the anticoagulation, thrombogenicity, leukocyte adherence, platelet adherence, endothelial cell damage repair, vessel wall contraction and vessel wall relaxation. They have the crucial role in the vascular homeostasis maintenance by promoting the formation of the new vessels and promote angiogenesis by paracrine effects. Endothelial dysfunction can lead to the disease condition like atherosclerosis, thrombosis, MI and chronic heart failure. Endothelial stem cell therapy has the potential role in all these disease conditions (Möbius-Winkler et al., 2009; Szmitko et al., 2003).

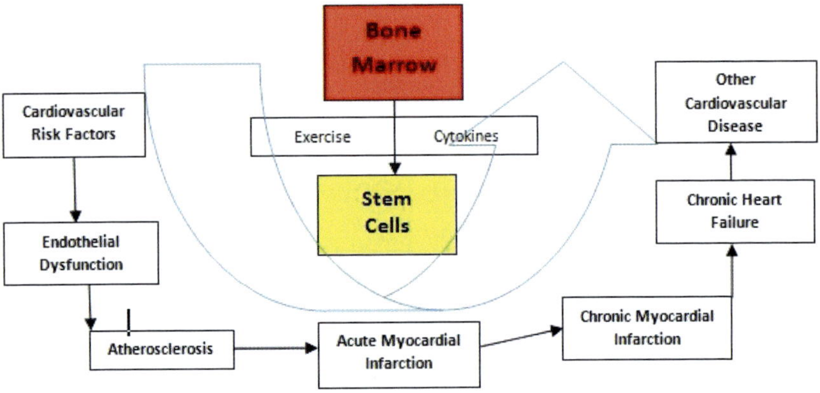

Figure 3: Therapeutic role of endothelial stem cells in various cardiovascular diseases (Möbius-Winkler et al., 2009).

Early phase clinical trials showed that endothelial stem cells therapy cause improvement in the exercise tolerance and improve in angina frequency (Lee and Poh, 2014).

One phase III clinical trial was also conducted to check the efficacy and safety of the endothelial stem cells therapy. However, the study was early terminated, due to no conclusion on the safety and efficacy was derived (Povsic et al., 2016).

3.6 Pluripotent stem cells (embryonic stem cells/induced pluripotent stem cells)

As mentioned in the introduction section, pluripotent cells have the capacity to differentiate into nearly all the cell type. So, pluripotent stem cell therapy has the great potential to repair myocardium injury (Chong and Murry, 2014).

Embryonic stem cells (ESCs) are developed from the early embryo however there are several concerns regarding usage of ESCs. Therapy with ESC requires the immunosuppressant, and it is not feasible to generate them from the patient's tissue with the properly standardized methods. Then after somatic cells reprogrammed to produce induced Pluripotent Stem Cells (iPSC) that has the capacity of self-renewal (Tanaka et al., 2015)

Pre-clinical studies showed that embryonic stem cell transplantation is feasible and it improves ventricular function in infracted failing hearts (Min et al., 2002; Chong and Murry, 2014). However, it requires further pre-clinical optimization (Ge et al., 2015). It has been reported that induced iPSC has the potential to induce a T-cell-dependent immune response. Therefore, the immunogenicity should be evaluated before any clinical application of these cells to the patients (Zhao et al., 2011).

4 Cardiac Stem Cells under Normal Conditions or Unstable Conditions

Cardiac myocyte cells death/apoptosis increases with increase in age. With advancement in the age, e.g., from 30 years to 60 years, approximately 85% of the original cardiac myocyte are lost. With the increase of age, myocyte replacement is also decreased. It has been reported that approximately 1% cardiac myocyte replacement can occur in the age of the 25 years and approximately 0.45% cardiac myocyte replacement can occur in the age of the 75 years (Leri et al., 2011).

There are two mechanisms proposed for the generation of the new cardiac myocyte. First is stem cell give rise to new cells and second is mature cell again re-enter to the mitotic cell cycle. However, overall turnover rate decreases evenly with age (Garbern and Lee, 2013).

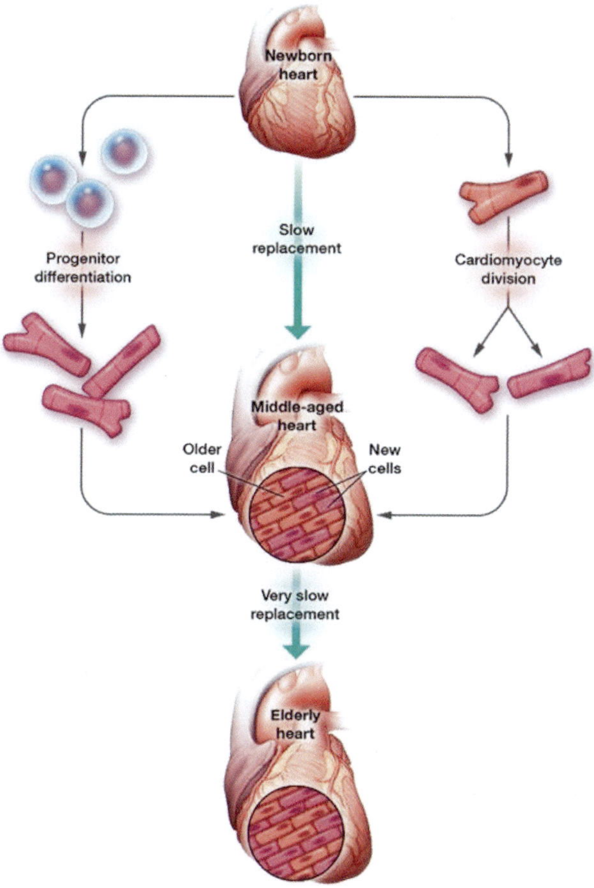

Figure 4: Proposed Mechanism of cardiogenesis under normal condition and aging

It has been proposed that cardiac myocyte involves in the repair process to compensate routine wear process. However, whenever extensive tissue damage occurs, e.g., in the conditions like MI, they are unable to compensate the loss (Leite et al., 2015).

Various theories have been proposed for the cardiac myocyte repair after injury (Figure 5). Generally, four theories have been proposed for the cardiac myocyte proliferation after the injury as described below (Garbern and Lee, 2013):

- Cardiac stem cell activation, proliferation and undergo differentiation that leads to new cardiac myocyte.
- Mature cardiac myocyte reenters the mitotic cell cycle; proliferation occurs that lead to new cardiac myocyte.
- Paracrine factors release such as various cytokines, growth factors, etc. to enhance the proliferation of the existing cardiac myocyte.
- Activation of the epicardium that leads to the development of the new blood vessels and that will also lead to new cardiac myocyte proliferation. Further, activation of the connective tissues, non-myocytes on the surface of the heart and surrounding epicardium also help the repair process of the cardiac myocyte.

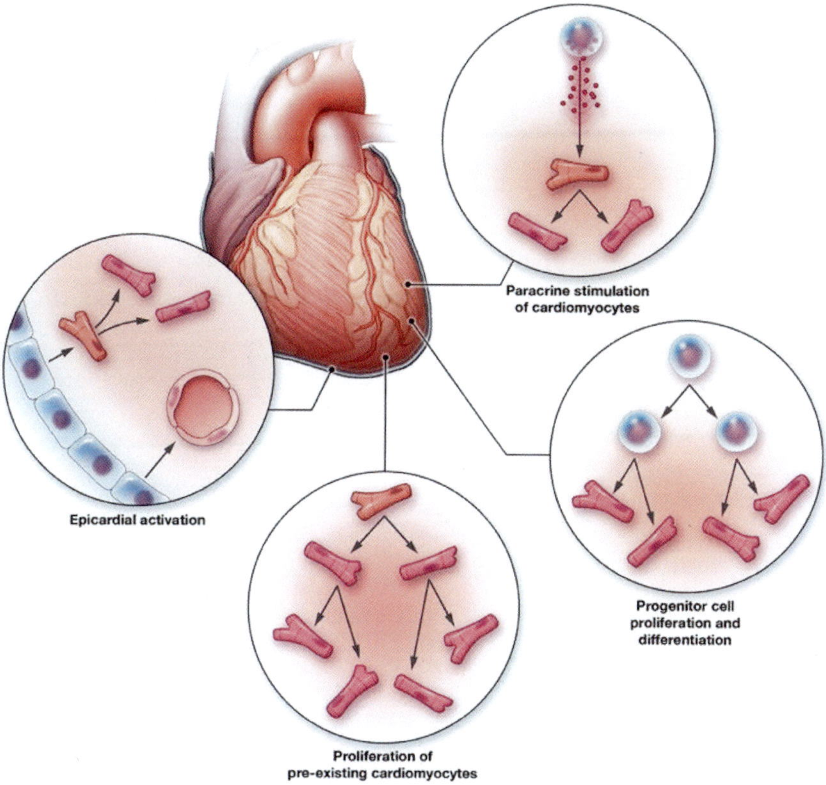

Figure 5: Proposed mechanisms for generation of new cardio-myocytes after injury (Garbern and Lee, 2013)

In few chronic disease conditions, such as diabetes, normal homeostasis of the cardiac stem cell becomes defective. In such situation cardiac cells gradually become non-differentiating and/or non-cyclic cells. So, the overall level of cardiac regeneration is not at the expected levels in the chronic disease state. This will gradually lead to the decompensated cardiac myopathy. In the condition of the excessive oxidative stress, there is a chance of cardiac stem cell impairment that will affect cardiac regenerative power, the poor contractile function of the heart and ultimately cardiac failure (Leite et al., 2015).

5 Cardiac Stem Cell Therapy

Various stem cell therapy e.g. cardiac and non-cardiac stem cells after transplantation can assist in the repair and can restore the previous cardiac contractile ability. Stem cells can be transplanted directly into a target organ and or administered peripherally with the help of various delivery routes. Broadly in the stem cell therapy, cardiac/extra-cardiac stem cells are isolated. These isolated cells (either endogenous cardiac stem cells/extra-cardiac stem cells) allows to expansion and differentiation in the appropriate *in-vitro* culture media. These cells are delivered to the cardiac myocyte with appropriate delivery mode. Then finally these stem cells through paracrine effects and trans-differentiation help (see the mechanism of action) in the myocyte generation and cardiac regeneration (Figure 6) (Mingling et al., 2011; Elam et al., 2013 and Faye et al., 2015). The main goals of the stem cells therapy are to have the selection of best cells, time of administration, selection of the delivery based on clinical trials performed. Safety of the patients needs to be ensured during the therapy. Till date there is no treatment in the market that involves stem cell therapy for the patients of the MI. However, results obtained from the various clinical trials with use of various stem cells are encouraging and require further investigation.

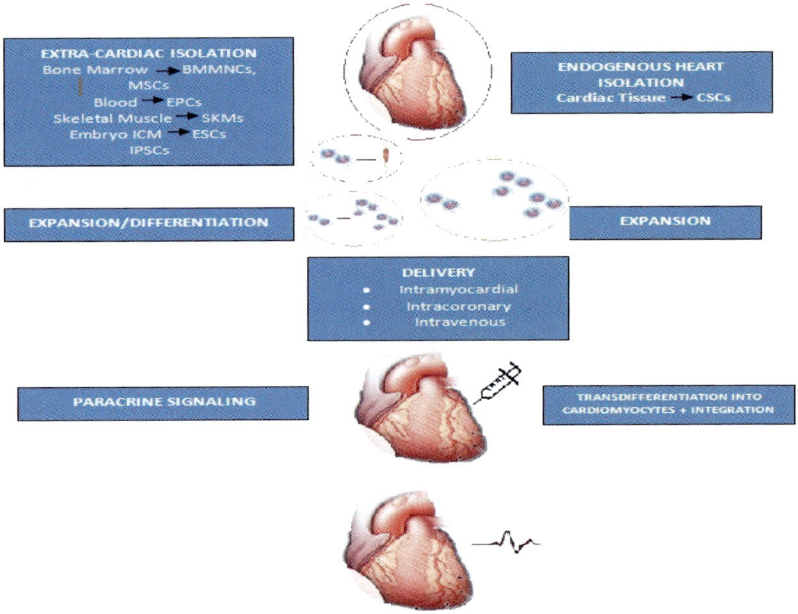

Figure 6: Schematic representation of events involved in regenerative stem cell treatment (Matar and Chong, 2014**).** BMMNC – Bone Marrow Mononuclear Cell, CSC – Cardiac Stem Cell, EPC – Endothelial Progenitor Cell, ESC – Embryonic Stem Cell, ICM – Inner Cell Mass, iPSC – Induced Pluripotent Stem Cell, MSC – Mesenchymal Stem Cell, SKM – Skeletal Myoblast

5.1 Stem cell - mechanisms of action

There are various stem direct or indirect mechanism are proposed in the literature by which stem cells therapy will help in the cardiac regeneration (Dimmeler et al., 2005; Gnecchi et al., 2008; Li et al., 2014)

- Delivered stem cells can be fused to the native cardiac myocyte to regenerate to compensate the lost myocardial cells.
- Delivered stem cells can proliferate and differentiated into the cardiac myocyte.
- Delivered stem cells can activate endogenous resident cardiac myocyte by various paracrine actions. These will promote growth and differentiation of the cardiac myocyte. Various paracrine factors include chemokine, cytokines and growth factors. Paracrine factors also inhibit cardiac apoptosis. Paracrine factors include plasminogen activator, insulin-like growth factor, vascular endothelial growth factor, interleukin-1, interleukin-6, fibroblast growth factor, adrenomedullin, etc. All these factors will promote the cardiac regeneration, cardiac remodeling neovascularization, and cardiac regeneration.

- Differentiation of stem cell to the endothelial cells, vascular smooth muscle cells, etc. to promote the neovascularization.

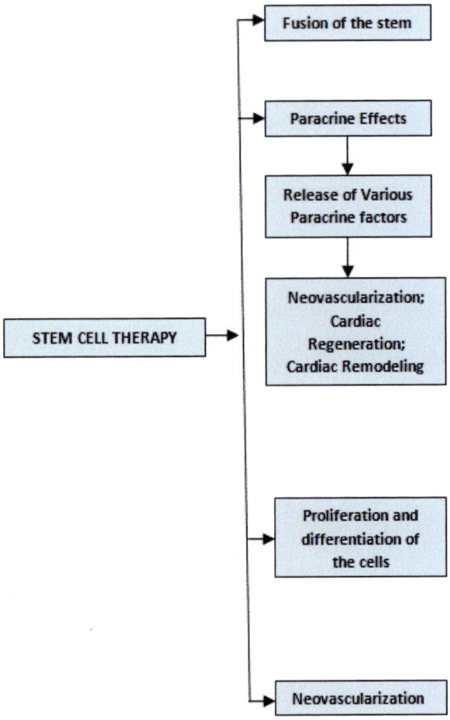

Figure 7: Possible Mechanisms of action of stem cell function

5.2 Cell delivery routes for cardiac stem cell therapy

Generally, there are three methods of delivery of transplanted cells; intra-myocardial (IM), intravenous (IV) and intracoronary (IC) delivery methods. The most clinically practiced form of the IC approach of cell delivery which is direct administration to myocardial sites via coronary artery. (Matar and Chong, 2014).

5.2.1 Intramuscular injection (IM)

With the help of the intramuscular injection, it is possible to inject the cells directly into the target area. Overall, donor cells can be directly injected into the myocardium.

5.2.1.1 Epicardial delivery

This procedure has been the precise, most direct, and accurate method for injecting various stem cells to an infracted / injured region of the heart. In this technique various techniques like ECHO (echocardiography), nuclear imaging etc. is utilized to identify the injured area before injecting the cells and also during the operation.

Delivery of the stem cells can be done during the right lateral mini thoracotomy or via open heart surgery like coronary artery bypass surgery (CABG). This technique though direct involves risk of invasive operation, and there will be greater chances of the complications like injection site perforation, arrhythmia, embolism and mortality (Sheng et al., 2013).

5.2.1.2 Endocardial delivery

In this delivery method, catheterization is done through the aortic valve and then stem cell injection is delivered to the endocardial surface in the perpendicular manner. This method is less invasive as compared with the epicardial method. A baseline 3D- the endocardial map is created which is color coded image of the heart. 'NOGA' system is created for the delivery of the stem cells. This system assists in identifying the target area. The catheter devices called named as Helix™, Myostar™, MyoCath™, and Stiletto™ can be used. (Campbell and Suzuki, 2012; Sherman et al., 2006 and Sheng et al., 2013).

5.2.1.3 Trans-coronary IM delivery

In this route of delivery, the stem cells can be delivered via percutaneous catheter via a coronary artery or coronary sinus. In this method, catheter is pass through the right atrium and cannulate the coronary sinus. This route of delivery has been successfully tested in the pre-clinically and few patients. This method is also less invasive like the endocardial method compared with epicardial method (Campbell and Suzuki, 2012; Sheng et al., 2013).

5.2.2 Intracoronary Injection

It is the method by which stem cell suspension is injected into the coronary circulation. In this method, coronary sinus blood vessels and coronary arteries are utilized for the stem cell transfer. This method has one of the advantages against the IM route. This method is less invasive i.e. associated less injury and delivery of stem cells will occur in a more physiological manner (Campbell and Suzuki, 2012).

It includes two approaches: 1) Antegrade Method and 2) Retrograde Method.

Antegrade Method: In this approach, the percutaneous catheter is passed through the femoral artery and targeted coronary artery is cannulated. Balloon is used to inflate coronary artery and then the stem cells are injected with high pressure. High pressure is used to prevent the backflow. After delivery of the stem cells, balloon is deflated to restore the normal flow. Major advantage of this technique is its familiriarity amoungst cardiologist (percutaneous technique). This method has minimal invasive nature and can be used in the high risk patient. Further complex mapping is not required as that in the IM route. Major drawback of this method is that cells cannot be deliver to the areas whose arterial supply is occluded (Campbell and Suzuki, 2012; Davies et al., 2016).

Retrograde method

As the name suggests this method target the femoral veins and not the femoral arteries. In this approach, the percutaneous catheter is passed through the **femoral veins** and then right atrium to cannulate the coronary sinus and target catheterizing the coronary vein. In this method also, cells are infused as mention above via high pressure. In contrast to antegrade method, there is less chance of coronary embolism and further stem cells can be delivered even though there is poor arterial supply (Campbell and Suzuki, 2012; Davies et al., 2016).

5.2.3 Intravenous (IV) Infusion

This is the minimally invasive and simple method amongst the methods described above. However, this method depends on the physiological signal from the injured heart, and this situation may not be present in a patient with heart failure. No. of cells reach to the target organ that is heart will depend on the blood flow rate to the cardiac tissues, and there are chances that they may deposit to the other organs (Davies et al., 2016).

5.3 Tissue engineering

Tissue engineering is the newer approach, and its focus is to regenerate the injured cardio-myocytes (Sheng et al., 2013).

In the tissue engineering strategies, biomaterials play a crucial role in facilitating cell transplantation. Biomaterial derived from the hydrogel includes collagen, fibrin, gelatin, etc. These are sourced from the natural environment and biocompatible. However, these cells have the less mechanical strength and contain the pathogen risk potential. Biomaterial derived from the synthetic material includes polyglycerol sebacate, poly-lactic-co-glycolic acid, poly-L-lactic acid, etc. This material is biocompatible and provide the mechanical strength. However, they may elicit the foreign response. This biomaterial allows cells to attach, migrate, differentiate and organize. The choice of cells is very crucial. The engineered cardiac tissue is prepared by culturing cells into the biomaterial and then transplanted to the MI heart. The ideal tissue generated should have the contractility ability, proliferate, differentiate, vascularize and electric transduction capacity (Alrefai et al., 2015; Tian et al., 2015).

6 Model For Predicting Coronary Artery Disease

By Dr. Bhargav Dave, PT, DPT & Dr. Myrtle Oates, MD

Risk Factors	Award 1 point for each applicable criteria	Total
Flow-Mediated Dilation (FMD) < 2% dilatation of Brachial Artery in response to increase in shear stress (Raitakari et al, 2000, Xu et al 2014 & Brevetti et al 2003)		
Asian / Diabetic / Age over 70 (Dave, B and Petrofksy J , 2016., Petrofsky et al, 2011, Petrofsky et at 2012, Petrofsky et at 2012, Petrofsky et at 2012)		
Endothelial derived microparticle (EMP) level over 0.303 $x 10^6$/ ml (Nozaki et al 2009)		
Smoker / Use of Tobacco		
Leptin Level over 25 ng/mL (Montazerifar et al, 2016)		
Total cholesterol mg/dL over LDL mg/dL ratio over 2.0 (Montazerifar et al, 2016)		
BMI over 25		
GRAND TOTAL		

Table 1: Any score over 5 represents higher risk of developing cardiovascular disease in subsequent decade

References

Akhtar, S. (2013). c-kit-positive cardiac stem cells as a potential candidate for heart repair, developments, challenges and future implications. *OA Stem Cells, 1*(1), 6.

Alrefai, M. T., Murali, D., Paul, A., Ridwan, K. M., Connell, J. M., & Shum-Tim, D. (2015). Cardiac tissue engineering and regeneration using cell-based therapy. *Stem Cells Cloning, 8*, 81-101. doi:10.2147/SCCAA.S54204

Andrae, J., Gallini, R., & Betsholtz, C. (2008). Role of platelet-derived growth factors in physiology and medicine. *Genes Dev, 22*(10), 1276-1312. doi:10.1101/gad.1653708

Arnous, S., Mozid, A., Martin, J., & Mathur, A. (2012). Bone marrow mononuclear cells and acute myocardial infarction. *Stem Cell Res Ther, 3*(1), 2. doi:10.1186/scrt93

B, H. B. A. S. (2011). Potency of Various Types of Stem Cells and their Transplantation. *J Stem Cell Res Ther, 1*(3), 1-6. doi:10.4172/2157-7633.1000115

Bailey, B., Fransioli, J., Gude, N. A., Alvarez, R., Jr., Zhang, X., Gustafsson, A. B., & Sussman, M. A. (2012). Sca-1 knockout impairs myocardial and cardiac progenitor cell function. *Circ Res, 111*(6), 750-760. doi:10.1161/CIRCRESAHA.112.274662

Bartunek, J., Behfar, A., Dolatabadi, D., Vanderheyden, M., Ostojic, M., Dens, J., . . . Terzic, A. (2013). Cardiopoietic stem cell therapy in heart failure: the C-CURE (Cardiopoietic stem Cell therapy in heart failURE) multicenter randomized trial with lineage-specified biologics. *J Am Coll Cardiol, 61*(23), 2329-2338. doi:10.1016/j.jacc.2013.02.071

Beltrami, A. P., Barlucchi, L., Torella, D., Baker, M., Limana, F., Chimenti, S., . . . Anversa, P. (2003). Adult cardiac stem cells are multipotent and support myocardial regeneration. *Cell, 114*(6), 763-776.

Bolli, R., Chugh, A. R., D'Amario, D., Loughran, J. H., Stoddard, M. F., Ikram, S., . . . Anversa, P. (2011). Cardiac stem cells in patients with ischaemic cardiomyopathy (SCIPIO): initial results of a randomised phase 1 trial. *Lancet, 378*(9806), 1847-1857. doi:10.1016/S0140-6736(11)61590-0

Brevetti, G., Silvestro, A., Schiano, V., & Chiariello, M. (2003). Endothelial dysfunction and cardiovascular risk prediction in peripheral arterial disease: additive value of flow-mediated dilation to ankle-brachial pressure index. *Circulation, 108*(17), 2093-2098. doi:10.1161/01.CIR.0000095273.92468.D9

Campbell, N. G., & Suzuki, K. (2012). Cell delivery routes for stem cell therapy to the heart: current and future approaches. *J Cardiovasc Transl Res, 5*(5), 713-726. doi:10.1007/s12265-012-9378-3

Chen, S. L., Fang, W. W., Ye, F., Liu, Y. H., Qian, J., Shan, S. J., . . . Sun, J. P. (2004). Effect on left ventricular function of intracoronary transplantation of autologous bone marrow mesenchymal stem cell in patients with acute myocardial infarction. *Am J Cardiol, 94*(1), 92-95. doi:10.1016/j.amjcard.2004.03.034

Chimenti, I., Smith, R. R., Li, T. S., Gerstenblith, G., Messina, E., Giacomello, A., & Marban, E. (2010). Relative roles of direct regeneration versus paracrine effects of human cardiosphere-derived cells transplanted into infarcted mice. *Circ Res, 106*(5), 971-980. doi:10.1161/CIRCRESAHA.109.210682

Chimenti, I., Smith, R. R., Li, T. S., Gerstenblith, G., Messina, E., Giacomello, A., & Marban, E. (2010). Relative roles of direct regeneration versus paracrine effects of human cardiosphere-derived cells transplanted into infarcted mice. *Circ Res, 106*(5), 971-980. doi:10.1161/CIRCRESAHA.109.210682

Choi, Y. H., Kurtz, A., & Stamm, C. (2011). Mesenchymal stem cells for cardiac cell therapy. *Hum Gene Ther, 22*(1), 3-17. doi:10.1089/hum.2010.211

Chong, J. J., & Murry, C. E. (2014). Cardiac regeneration using pluripotent stem cells--progression to large animal models. *Stem Cell Res, 13*(3 Pt B), 654-665. doi:10.1016/j.scr.2014.06.005

Chong, J. J., Reinecke, H., Iwata, M., Torok-Storb, B., Stempien-Otero, A., & Murry, C. E. (2013). Progenitor cells identified by PDGFR-alpha expression in the developing and diseased human heart. *Stem Cells Dev, 22*(13), 1932-1943. doi:10.1089/scd.2012.0542

Cordero, D. R., Brugmann, S., Chu, Y., Bajpai, R., Jame, M., & Helms, J. A. (2011). Cranial neural crest cells on the move: their roles in craniofacial development. *Am J Med*

Genet A, 155A(2), 270-279. doi:10.1002/ajmg.a.33702

Dave, B. (2016). Bioresorbable Scaffolds: Current Evidences in the Treatment of Coronary Artery Disease. *Journal of Clinical and Diagnostic Research, 10*(10), OE01-OE07. doi:10.7860/JCDR/2016/21915.8429

Dave, B. (2016). Recanalization of Chronic Total Occlusion Lesions: A Critical Appraisal of Current Devices and Techniques. *Journal of Clinical and Diagnostic Research, 10*(09), E1-E7. doi:10.7860/JCDR/2016/21853.8396

Dave, B. P., J. (2016). *Heat and Human Interaction* (1st ed. Vol. 1). Texas, United States of America: Srinivas University Press.

Davies, N. G., K; Ngoepe, M; Franz, T; Lecour, S. (2016). Delivery Modes for Cardiac Stem Cell Therapy. *Stem Cells and Cardiac Regeneration, R. Madonna*, 165-190.

Dawn, B., Stein, A. B., Urbanek, K., Rota, M., Whang, B., Rastaldo, R., . . . Bolli, R. (2005). Cardiac stem cells delivered intravascularly traverse the vessel barrier, regenerate infarcted myocardium, and improve cardiac function. *Proc Natl Acad Sci U S A, 102*(10), 3766-3771. doi:10.1073/pnas.0405957102

Dimmeler, S., Zeiher, A. M., & Schneider, M. D. (2005). Unchain my heart: the scientific foundations of cardiac repair. *J Clin Invest, 115*(3), 572-583. doi:10.1172/JCI24283

Elhami, E., Dietz, B., Xiang, B., Deng, J., Wang, F., Chi, C., . . .

Tian, G. (2013). Assessment of three techniques for delivering stem cells to the heart using PET and MR imaging. *EJNMMI Res, 3*(1), 72. doi:10.1186/2191-219X-3-72

Feyen, D. A., Gaetani, R., Doevendans, P. A., & Sluijter, J. P. (2016). Stem cell-based therapy: Improving myocardial cell delivery. *Adv Drug Deliv Rev*. doi:10.1016/j.addr.2016.04.023

Garbern, J. C., & Lee, R. T. (2013). Cardiac stem cell therapy and the promise of heart regeneration. *Cell Stem Cell, 12*(6), 689-698. doi:10.1016/j.stem.2013.05.008

Gardner, R. L. (2002). Human experimental chimaerism: Chimaeras as a source of stem cells. *Reprod Biomed Online, 5*(2), 103.

Gardner, R. L. (2002). Stem cells: potency, plasticity and public perception. *J Anat, 200*(Pt 3), 277-282.

Ge, Z. L., S; Le, T; Remedios, C; Chong J. (2015). Cardiac stem cells: translation to human studies. *Biophys Rev, 7*, 127-139. doi:10.1007/s12551-014-0148-0

Gittenberger-de Groot, A. C., Winter, E. M., & Poelmann, R. E. (2010). Epicardium-derived cells (EPDCs) in development, cardiac disease and repair of ischemia. *J Cell Mol Med, 14*(5), 1056-1060. doi:10.1111/j.1582-4934.2010.01077.x

Gnecchi, M., Zhang, Z., Ni, A., & Dzau, V. J. (2008). Paracrine mechanisms in adult stem cell signaling and therapy. *Circ Res, 103*(11), 1204-1219.

doi:10.1161/CIRCRESAHA.108.176826

Hare, J. M., Fishman, J. E., Gerstenblith, G., DiFede Velazquez, D. L., Zambrano, J. P., Suncion, V. Y., . . . Lardo, A. (2012). Comparison of allogeneic vs autologous bone marrow-derived mesenchymal stem cells delivered by transendocardial injection in patients with ischemic cardiomyopathy: the POSEIDON randomized trial. *JAMA, 308*(22), 2369-2379. doi:10.1001/jama.2012.25321

Hierlihy, A. M., Seale, P., Lobe, C. G., Rudnicki, M. A., & Megeney, L. A. (2002). The post-natal heart contains a myocardial stem cell population. *FEBS Lett, 530*(1-3), 239-243.

Hima Bindu, A. S., B. (2011). Potency of Various Types of Stem Cells and their Transplantation. *J Stem Cell Res The, 1*(3), 6.

Holmes, C., & Stanford, W. L. (2007). Concise review: stem cell antigen-1: expression, function, and enigma. *Stem Cells, 25*(6), 1339-1347. doi:10.1634/stemcells.2006-0644

Karantalis, V., DiFede, D. L., Gerstenblith, G., Pham, S., Symes, J., Zambrano, J. P., . . . Hare, J. M. (2014). Autologous mesenchymal stem cells produce concordant improvements in regional function, tissue perfusion, and fibrotic burden when administered to patients undergoing coronary artery bypass grafting: The Prospective Randomized Study of Mesenchymal Stem Cell Therapy in Patients Undergoing Cardiac Surgery (PROMETHEUS) trial. *Circ Res, 114*(8), 1302-1310.

doi:10.1161/CIRCRESAHA.114.303180

Karantalis, V., & Hare, J. M. (2015). Use of mesenchymal stem cells for therapy of cardiac disease. *Circ Res, 116*(8), 1413-1430. doi:10.1161/CIRCRESAHA.116.303614

Kumar, L., Ganessan, P., Ghosh, I., Panda, D., Gogia, A., & Mandhania, S. (2010). Autologous blood stem cell transplantation for Hodgkin and non-Hodgkin lymphoma: complications and outcome. *Natl Med J India, 23*(6), 330-335.

Kumar, R., Sharma, A., Pattnaik, A. K., & Varadwaj, P. K. (2010). Stem cells: An overview with respect to cardiovascular and renal disease. *J Nat Sci Biol Med, 1*(1), 43-52. doi:10.4103/0976-9668.71674

Laflamme, M. A., & Murry, C. E. (2011). Heart regeneration. *Nature, 473*(7347), 326-335. doi:10.1038/nature10147

Laugwitz, K. L., Moretti, A., Caron, L., Nakano, A., & Chien, K. R. (2008). Islet1 cardiovascular progenitors: a single source for heart lineages? *Development, 135*(2), 193-205. doi:10.1242/dev.001883

Le, T., & Chong, J. (2016). Cardiac progenitor cells for heart repair. *Cell Death Discov, 2*, 16052. doi:10.1038/cddiscovery.2016.52

Lee, P. S., & Poh, K. K. (2014). Endothelial progenitor cells in cardiovascular diseases. *World J Stem Cells, 6*(3), 355-366. doi:10.4252/wjsc.v6.i3.355

Leite, C. F., Almeida, T. R., Lopes, C. S., & Dias da Silva, V. J. (2015). Multipotent stem cells of the heart-do they have therapeutic promise? *Front Physiol, 6*, 123. doi:10.3389/fphys.2015.00123

Leri, A., Kajstura, J., & Anversa, P. (2011). Role of cardiac stem cells in cardiac pathophysiology: a paradigm shift in human myocardial biology. *Circ Res, 109*(8), 941-961. doi:10.1161/CIRCRESAHA.111.243154

Leri, A., Rota, M., Hosoda, T., Goichberg, P., & Anversa, P. (2014). Cardiac stem cell niches. *Stem Cell Res, 13*(3 Pt B), 631-646. doi:10.1016/j.scr.2014.09.001

Li, N., Wang, C., Jia, L., & Du, J. (2014). Heart regeneration, stem cells, and cytokines. *Regen Med Res, 2*(1), 6. doi:10.1186/2050-490X-2-6

Li, T. S., Cheng, K., Malliaras, K., Smith, R. R., Zhang, Y., Sun, B., . . . Marban, E. (2012). Direct comparison of different stem cell types and subpopulations reveals superior paracrine potency and myocardial repair efficacy with cardiosphere-derived cells. *J Am Coll Cardiol, 59*(10), 942-953. doi:10.1016/j.jacc.2011.11.029

Makkar, R. R., Smith, R. R., Cheng, K., Malliaras, K., Thomson, L. E., Berman, D., . . . Marban, E. (2012). Intracoronary cardiosphere-derived cells for heart regeneration after myocardial infarction (CADUCEUS): a prospective, randomised phase 1 trial. *Lancet, 379*(9819), 895-904. doi:10.1016/S0140-6736(12)60195-0

Matar, A. A., & Chong, J. J. (2014). Stem cell therapy for cardiac dysfunction. *Springerplus, 3*, 440. doi:10.1186/2193-1801-3-440

Menasche, P., Hagege, A. A., Vilquin, J. T., Desnos, M., Abergel, E., Pouzet, B., . . . Duboc, D. (2003). Autologous skeletal myoblast transplantation for severe postinfarction left ventricular dysfunction. *J Am Coll Cardiol, 41*(7), 1078-1083.

Min, J. Y., Yang, Y., Converso, K. L., Liu, L., Huang, Q., Morgan, J. P., & Xiao, Y. F. (2002). Transplantation of embryonic stem cells improves cardiac function in postinfarcted rats. *J Appl Physiol (1985), 92*(1), 288-296.

Mingliang, R., Bo, Z., & Zhengguo, W. (2011). Stem cells for cardiac repair: status, mechanisms, and new strategies. *Stem Cells Int, 2011*, 310928. doi:10.4061/2011/310928

Miyamoto, S., Kawaguchi, N., Ellison, G. M., Matsuoka, R., Shin'oka, T., & Kurosawa, H. (2010). Characterization of long-term cultured c-kit+ cardiac stem cells derived from adult rat hearts. *Stem Cells Dev, 19*(1), 105-116. doi:10.1089/scd.2009.0041

Mobius-Winkler, S., Hollriegel, R., Schuler, G., & Adams, V. (2009). Endothelial progenitor cells: implications for cardiovascular disease. *Cytometry A, 75*(1), 25-37. doi:10.1002/cyto.a.20669

Montazerifar, F., Bolouri, A., Paghalea, R. S., Mahani, M. K., & Karajibani, M. (2016). Obesity, Serum Resistin and Leptin Levels Linked to Coronary Artery Disease. *Arq Bras Cardiol*, 0. doi:10.5935/abc.20160134

Moretti, A., Caron, L., Nakano, A., Lam, J. T., Bernshausen, A., Chen, Y., . . . Chien, K. R. (2006). Multipotent embryonic isl1+ progenitor cells lead to cardiac, smooth muscle, and endothelial cell diversification. *Cell, 127*(6), 1151-1165. doi:10.1016/j.cell.2006.10.029

Mouquet, F., Pfister, O., Jain, M., Oikonomopoulos, A., Ngoy, S., Summer, R., . . . Liao, R. (2005). Restoration of cardiac progenitor cells after myocardial infarction by self-proliferation and selective homing of bone marrow-derived stem cells. *Circ Res, 97*(11), 1090-1092. doi:10.1161/01.RES.0000194330.66545.f5

Nozaki, T., Sugiyama, S., Koga, H., Sugamura, K., Ohba, K., Matsuzawa, Y., . . . Ogawa, H. (2009). Significance of a multiple biomarkers strategy including endothelial dysfunction to improve risk stratification for cardiovascular events in patients at high risk for coronary heart disease. *J Am Coll Cardiol, 54*(7), 601-608. doi:10.1016/j.jacc.2009.05.022

Orlic, D., Kajstura, J., Chimenti, S., Bodine, D. M., Leri, A., & Anversa, P. (2003). Bone marrow stem cells regenerate infarcted myocardium. *Pediatr Transplant, 7 Suppl 3*, 86-88.

Oyama, T., Nagai, T., Wada, H., Naito, A. T., Matsuura, K., Iwanaga, K., . . . Komuro, I. (2007). Cardiac side population cells have a potential to migrate and differentiate into cardiomyocytes in vitro and in vivo. *J Cell Biol, 176*(3), 329-341. doi:10.1083/jcb.200603014

Petrofsky, J., Alshahmmari, F., Yim, J. E., Hamdan, A., Lee, H., Neupane, S., . . . Desai, R. (2011). The interrealtionship between locally applied heat, ageing and skin blood flow on heat transfer into and from the skin. *J Med Eng*

Technol, 35(5), 262-274. doi:10.3109/03091902.2011.580039

Petrofsky, J., Berk, L., Alshammari, F., Lee, H., Hamdan, A., Yim, J. E., . . . Al-Nakhli, H. (2012). The effect of moist air on skin blood flow and temperature in subjects with and without diabetes. *Diabetes Technol Ther, 14*(2), 105-116. doi:10.1089/dia.2011.0128

Petrofsky, J. S., Alshahmmari, F., Lee, H., Hamdan, A., Yim, J. E., Shetye, G., . . . Desai, R. (2012). Reduced endothelial function in the skin in Southeast Asians compared to Caucasians. *Med Sci Monit, 18*(1), CR1-8.

Petrofsky, J. S., Berk, L., Alshammari, F., Lee, H., Hamdan, A., Yim, J. E., . . . Al-Nakhli, H. (2012). The interrelationship between air temperature and humidity as applied locally to the skin: the resultant response on skin temperature and blood flow with age differences. *Med Sci Monit, 18*(4), CR201-208.

Pfister, O., Oikonomopoulos, A., Sereti, K. I., Sohn, R. L., Cullen, D., Fine, G. C., . . . Liao, R. (2008). Role of the ATP-binding cassette transporter Abcg2 in the phenotype and function of cardiac side population cells. *Circ Res, 103*(8), 825-835. doi:10.1161/CIRCRESAHA.108.174615

Pittenger, M. F., & Martin, B. J. (2004). Mesenchymal stem cells and their potential as cardiac therapeutics. *Circ Res, 95*(1), 9-20. doi:10.1161/01.RES.0000135902.99383.6f

Ponten, A., Li, X., Thoren, P., Aase, K., Sjoblom, T., Ostman,

A., & Eriksson, U. (2003). Transgenic overexpression of platelet-derived growth factor-C in the mouse heart induces cardiac fibrosis, hypertrophy, and dilated cardiomyopathy. *Am J Pathol, 163*(2), 673-682. doi:10.1016/S0002-9440(10)63694-2

Povsic, T. J., Henry, T. D., Traverse, J. H., Fortuin, F. D., Schaer, G. L., Kereiakes, D. J., . . . Investigators, R. (2016). The RENEW Trial: Efficacy and Safety of Intramyocardial Autologous CD34(+) Cell Administration in Patients With Refractory Angina. *JACC Cardiovasc Interv, 9*(15), 1576-1585. doi:10.1016/j.jcin.2016.05.003

Raitakari, O. T., & Celermajer, D. S. (2000). Flow-mediated dilatation. *Br J Clin Pharmacol, 50*(5), 397-404.

Satessa, G., Lenjisa, J., Gebremariam, E., Woldu, M. (2015). Stem Cell Therapy for Myocardial Infarction: Challenges and Prospects. *Journal of Stem Cell Research & Therapy, 5*(3), 5. doi:10.4172/2157-7633.1000270

Sheng, C. C., Zhou, L., & Hao, J. (2013). Current stem cell delivery methods for myocardial repair. *Biomed Res Int, 2013*, 547902. doi:10.1155/2013/547902

Sherman, W., Martens, T. P., Viles-Gonzalez, J. F., & Siminiak, T. (2006). Catheter-based delivery of cells to the heart. *Nat Clin Pract Cardiovasc Med, 3 Suppl 1*, S57-64. doi:10.1038/ncpcardio0446

Sieber-Blum, M. (2004). Cardiac neural crest stem cells. *Anat Rec A Discov Mol Cell Evol Biol, 276*(1), 34-42. doi:10.1002/ar.a.10132

Simari, R. D., Pepine, C. J., Traverse, J. H., Henry, T. D., Bolli, R., Spoon, D. B., . . . Moye, L. A. (2014). Bone marrow mononuclear cell therapy for acute myocardial infarction: a perspective from the cardiovascular cell therapy research network. *Circ Res, 114*(10), 1564-1568. doi:10.1161/CIRCRESAHA.114.303720

Sun, Y., Liang, X., Najafi, N., Cass, M., Lin, L., Cai, C. L., . . . Evans, S. M. (2007). Islet 1 is expressed in distinct cardiovascular lineages, including pacemaker and coronary vascular cells. *Dev Biol, 304*(1), 286-296. doi:10.1016/j.ydbio.2006.12.048

Szmitko, P. E., Fedak, P. W., Weisel, R. D., Stewart, D. J., Kutryk, M. J., & Verma, S. (2003). Endothelial progenitor cells: new hope for a broken heart. *Circulation, 107*(24), 3093-3100. doi:10.1161/01.CIR.0000074242.66719.4A

Tanaka, A., Yuasa, S., Node, K., & Fukuda, K. (2015). Cardiovascular Disease Modeling Using Patient-Specific Induced Pluripotent Stem Cells. *Int J Mol Sci, 16*(8), 18894-18922. doi:10.3390/ijms160818894

Taylor, D. A., Atkins, B. Z., Hungspreugs, P., Jones, T. R., Reedy, M. C., Hutcheson, K. A., . . . Kraus, W. E. (1998). Regenerating functional myocardium: improved performance after skeletal myoblast transplantation. *Nat Med, 4*(8), 929-933.

The Lancet, E. (2014). Expression of concern: the SCIPIO trial. *Lancet, 383*(9925), 1279. doi:10.1016/S0140-6736(14)60608-5

Tian, S., Liu, Q., Gnatovskiy, L., Ma, P. X., & Wang, Z. (2015).

Heart Regeneration with Embryonic Cardiac Progenitor Cells and Cardiac Tissue Engineering. *J Stem Cell Transplant Biol, 1*(1). doi:10.19104/jstb.2015.104

Unno, K., Jain, M., & Liao, R. (2012). Cardiac side population cells: moving toward the center stage in cardiac regeneration. *Circ Res, 110*(10), 1355-1363. doi:10.1161/CIRCRESAHA.111.243014

van Berlo, J. H., Kanisicak, O., Maillet, M., Vagnozzi, R. J., Karch, J., Lin, S. C., . . . Molkentin, J. D. (2014). c-kit+ cells minimally contribute cardiomyocytes to the heart. *Nature, 509*(7500), 337-341. doi:10.1038/nature13309

Veltman, C. E., Soliman, O. I., Geleijnse, M. L., Vletter, W. B., Smits, P. C., ten Cate, F. J., . . . van der Giessen, W. J. (2008). Four-year follow-up of treatment with intramyocardial skeletal myoblasts injection in patients with ischaemic cardiomyopathy. *Eur Heart J, 29*(11), 1386-1396. doi:10.1093/eurheartj/ehn171

Wang, X., Hu, Q., Nakamura, Y., Lee, J., Zhang, G., From, A. H., & Zhang, J. (2006). The role of the sca-1+/CD31- cardiac progenitor cell population in postinfarction left ventricular remodeling. *Stem Cells, 24*(7), 1779-1788. doi:10.1634/stemcells.2005-0386

Weeke-Klimp, A., Bax, N. A., Bellu, A. R., Winter, E. M., Vrolijk, J., Plantinga, J., . . . Lie-Venema, H. (2010). Epicardium-derived cells enhance proliferation, cellular maturation and alignment of cardiomyocytes. *J Mol Cell Cardiol, 49*(4), 606-616. doi:10.1016/j.yjmcc.2010.07.007

White, I. A., Sanina, C., Balkan, W., & Hare, J. M. (2016). Mesenchymal Stem Cells in Cardiology. *Methods Mol Biol, 1416*, 55-87. doi:10.1007/978-1-4939-3584-0_4

Williams, A. R., & Hare, J. M. (2011). Mesenchymal stem cells: biology, pathophysiology, translational findings, and therapeutic implications for cardiac disease. *Circ Res, 109*(8), 923-940. doi:10.1161/CIRCRESAHA.111.243147

Winter, E. M., & Gittenberger-de Groot, A. C. (2007). Epicardium-derived cells in cardiogenesis and cardiac regeneration. *Cell Mol Life Sci, 64*(6), 692-703. doi:10.1007/s00018-007-6522-3

Winter, E. M., Grauss, R. W., Hogers, B., van Tuyn, J., van der Geest, R., Lie-Venema, H., . . . Gittenberger-de Groot, A. C. (2007). Preservation of left ventricular function and attenuation of remodeling after transplantation of human epicardium-derived cells into the infarcted mouse heart. *Circulation, 116*(8), 917-927. doi:10.1161/CIRCULATIONAHA.106.668178

Xu, Y., Arora, R. C., Hiebert, B. M., Lerner, B., Szwajcer, A., McDonald, K., . . . Tangri, N. (2014). Non-invasive endothelial function testing and the risk of adverse outcomes: a systematic review and meta-analysis. *Eur Heart J Cardiovasc Imaging, 15*(7), 736-746. doi:10.1093/ehjci/jet256

Zhao, T., Zhang, Z. N., Rong, Z., & Xu, Y. (2011). Immunogenicity of induced pluripotent stem cells. *Nature, 474*(7350), 212-215. doi:10.1038/nature10135

The Mother's Symbol

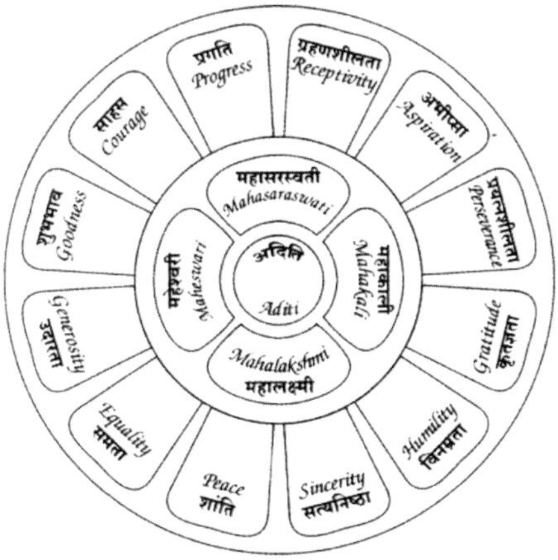

श्री माताजीका प्रतीक

The Mother's Symbol

- **Sincerity:**
  To be constantly the true flame that burns like an offering.
- **Humility:**
  We are nothing in ourselves.
- **Gratitude:**
  The whole being offers itself to the Lord in absolute trust.
- **Perseverance :**
  The decision to go to the very end.
- **Aspiration:**
  We must aspire with all our being for the manifestation to come soon and complete.
- **Receptivity:**
  The whole being is aware of the Divine Will and obeys it.

- **Progress:**
  The will for progress by the urge towards perfection.
- **Courage:**
  When we trust in the Divine Grace we get an unfailing courage.
- ▪ **Goodness:**
  Good is all that helps the individual and the world towards their Divine Fullness.
- **Generosity:**
  Gives and gives oneself without bargaining.
- ▪ **Equality:**
  The Supreme Divine Nature is founded on equality.
- **Peace:**
  The Divine is Supreme Peace. Be with the Divine and you will be in peace.

• *The Mother* ▪ *Sri Aurobindo*

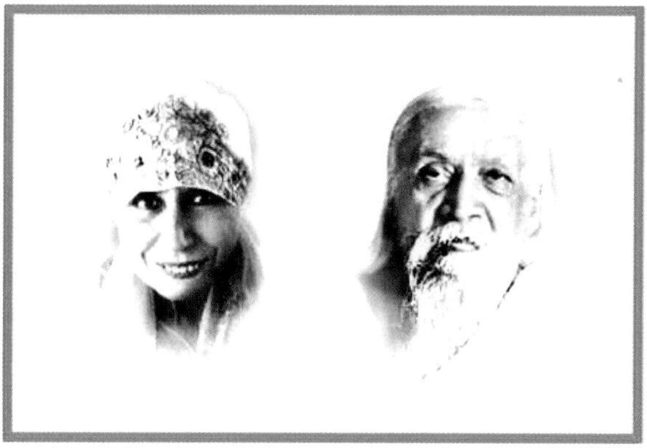

Divine Mother & Maharshi Aurobindo